DECODING ADHD

Finding Solutions For Your Child's Unique Needs

I0449240

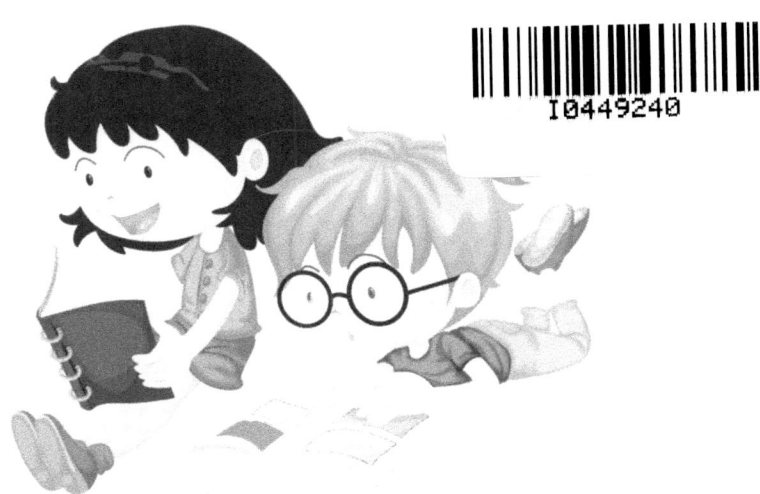

Dr. A. Anish

Copyright ©2023 Dr. A. Anish

All rights reserved.
No Part of this book may be reproduced or stored in a retrieval system, or transmitted in any form or by any means, electronic, mechanical, photocopying, recording, or otherwise, without express written permission of the author.

FOREWORD

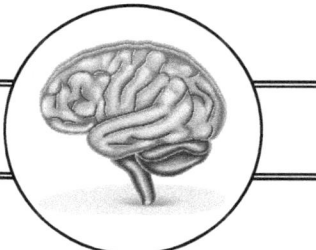

Dear readers,

I am delighted to introduce to you a revolutionary guide in the field of ADHD management. As a parent myself, I understand the challenges that come with raising a child with ADHD. And no doubt, you too have experienced the same exasperation, fatigue and feelings of hopelessness. But, I assure you that this book is here to bring hope, support and practical strategies in understanding what ADHD is and how you can manage it in your child.

ADHD is not just about the inability to focus, impulsivity and hyperactivity; it is a complex neurological condition that requires a multifaceted approach to management. In this book, you will learn about the biological, psychological and environmental factors that contribute to ADHD. Moreover, you will be provided with evidence-based strategies that have been proven effective in managing ADHD.

This guide is not just for parents, but for anyone who is involved in managing ADHD. It is written in a clear, concise and accessible manner that makes it easy to follow and implement the strategies provided. I am confident that you will find this guide to be an invaluable resource that will help transform the life of your child positively.

In conclusion, I would like to say that there is no need to feel powerless when it comes to managing ADHD. With the right knowledge and understanding, we can help our children with ADHD reach their full potential. So, let's get started on this journey together.

Best regards,
Jane Rowling

PREFACE

Attention Deficit Hyperactivity Disorder (ADHD) is a neurodevelopmental disorder that affects millions of people worldwide. It is a disorder that often begins in childhood, and if left untreated, can have severe consequences on an individual's social, emotional, and academic success. As someone who has experienced the challenges of ADHD, I have learned firsthand how crucial it is to understand the disorder and find ways to manage its symptoms.

Through my personal journey and research, I have compiled this book to help individuals with ADHD and their loved ones to better understand the disorder and learn effective strategies for managing its symptoms. This book will provide insight into the various aspects of ADHD, the symptoms, and the diagnostic process. More importantly, it will offer practical tips and techniques proven to help manage ADHD symptoms in various facets of life, from school to work, and daily personal life.

The purpose of this book is to empower individuals with ADHD and their loved ones to gain a deeper understanding of the disorder and provide them with the tools to manage their symptoms confidently. Whether you are an individual with ADHD or a parent, teacher, or friend of someone with ADHD, this book is designed to help you navigate the challenges of ADHD and achieve success.

INTRODUCTION

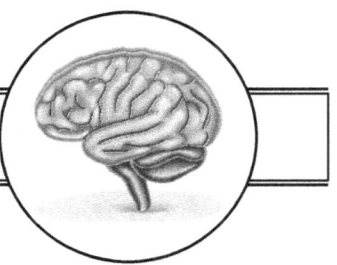

Attention Deficit Hyperactivity Disorder (ADHD) is a neurodevelopmental disorder that affects both children and adults. It is a complex condition that can cause difficulty in paying attention, impulsivity, and hyperactivity. Children with ADHD often face difficulties in concentration, following rules, and completing tasks, leading to poor school performance and relationship problems. As parents, watching your child struggle with ADHD can be a daunting experience. However, with the right strategies and support, managing your child's ADHD can become an empowering and successful journey.

In this book, we will explore what ADHD is and how it affects children. We will discuss different types of ADHD, along with their symptoms and diagnostic criteria. Additionally, we will cover the various tools and techniques that can help parents successfully manage their child's ADHD, including behavioural and lifestyle changes, therapy, medication and special education services.

This book aims to empower parents with the tools and knowledge to support their children with ADHD. Whether you're a parent new to the condition or have been managing it for a while, this book will provide practical and effective solutions to support your child, leading to better performance in school and at home. Let's get started on this journey together.

TABLE OF CONTENTS

Chapters

CHAPTER ONE

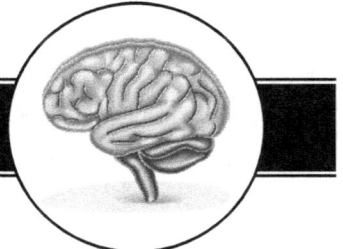

INTRODUCTION: UNDERSTANDING ADHD, ITS PREVALENCE, AND ITS IMPACT ON CHILDREN

Attention Deficit Hyperactivity Disorder (ADHD) is a neurodevelopmental disorder that affects a significant number of children worldwide. It is characterized by inattention, hyperactivity, and impulsivity, which can impair a child's ability to learn, socialize, and function in daily life.

According to the Centers for Disease Control and Prevention (CDC), approximately 6.1 million children aged 2-17 years in the United States have been diagnosed with ADHD, which accounts for around 9.4% of all children. This prevalence has been steadily increasing over the years, and research suggests that ADHD can be traced back to childhood and persists into adulthood for many individuals.

The impact of ADHD on children can be far-reaching and can affect various areas of their lives, including academic, social, and emotional functioning. Children with ADHD may experience difficulty paying attention in class, completing schoolwork, organizing tasks, following rules, making friends, and controlling their behavior.

In school, children with ADHD may struggle to meet academic expectations, leading to poor grades, reduced self-esteem, and increased risk of dropping out. They may also experience social rejection, which can further exacerbate their difficulties with peer relationships and impact their overall wellbeing.

ADHD can also affect a child's emotional functioning, as they may struggle with low self-esteem, anxiety, and depression. These emotional challenges can persist into adulthood, leading to difficulties with employment, relationships, and overall life satisfaction.

In conclusion, ADHD is a prevalent disorder that affects many children across the world. Its impact on children can be severe and far-reaching, leading to academic, social, and emotional difficulties. Recognizing the signs and symptoms of ADHD early on and seeking appropriate treatment can significantly improve a child's life outcomes and overall wellbeing.

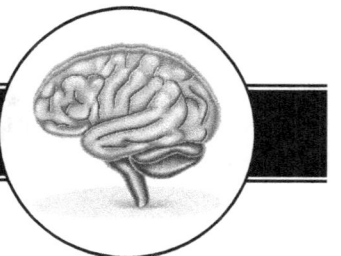

CHAPTER TWO

WHAT IS ADHD? SYMPTOMS, DIAGNOSIS, AND CAUSES

Attention deficit hyperactivity disorder (ADHD) is a neurodevelopmental disorder that affects people of all ages, genders, and races. It is characterized by inattention, hyperactivity, and impulsivity, which makes it difficult for individuals to focus on tasks, regulate their behavior, and control their emotions. In this article, we will delve into the symptoms, diagnosis, and causes of ADHD.

Symptoms

The symptoms of ADHD vary from person to person, but they generally fall into two categories: inattention and hyperactivity/impulsivity. People with ADHD may experience some or all of the symptoms below:

Inattention:

- Difficulty in sustaining attention on tasks or activities
- Difficulty organizing tasks and activities
- Easily distracted by external stimuli
- Forgetful in daily activities
- Avoiding or disliking work that requires sustained mental effort
- Losing things necessary for tasks and activities

Hyperactivity/Impulsivity:
- Fidgeting or squirming in their seat
- Excessive talking or interrupting conversations
- Difficulty playing or doing leisure activities quietly
- Difficulty waiting their turn
- Frequently leaving their seat in situations where sitting is expected
- Acting as if they are "on the go" or "driven by a motor"

Diagnosis

Diagnosing ADHD can be a complex process, as the symptoms can mimic other disorders, such as anxiety, depression, or learning disabilities. There is no one definitive diagnostic test for ADHD, so the diagnosis is usually made based on a combination of factors, which may include:

- Interviews with the individual and their family members
- Behavioral observations in different settings (e.g., home, school, and work)
- Psychological testing to rule out other diagnoses
- Rating scales completed by the individual, family members, and teachers
- Medical evaluation to rule out any physical health concerns

It is important to note that only a licensed healthcare professional, such as a psychiatrist or psychologist, can diagnose ADHD. Self-diagnosis or relying on the advice of non-professionals is not recommended.

Causes

The exact causes of ADHD are not fully understood, but research has indicated that genetics, brain structure and function, and environmental factors may play a role.

While the causes of ADHD are not entirely known, there are several factors that can contribute to the development of this condition.

1. Genetics

Numerous studies have suggested that genetics play a crucial role in the development of ADHD. If one or both parents have ADHD, there is a higher likelihood of their children inheriting the condition. According to research, up to 80% of children with ADHD have a close relative with the disorder.

2. Brain Function
Studies suggest that differences in how the brain functions may also contribute to ADHD. Neurotransmitters, such as dopamine and norepinephrine, are responsible for regulating attention, and individuals with ADHD may have an imbalance in these chemical messengers. Another area of the brain that may impact ADHD is the frontal lobe, which is responsible for inhibiting impulses and decision making.

3. Environmental Factors
Environmental factors, such as exposure to toxins, alcohol or tobacco use during pregnancy, premature delivery, low birth weight, and brain injury, can increase the risk of developing ADHD. Additionally, children growing up in chaotic or abusive environments may also have a higher likelihood of developing ADHD.

4. Diet
Some studies suggest that diet may play a role in the development of ADHD. Consuming high amounts of processed foods with artificial flavors and colors, sugar, and preservatives may exacerbate symptoms of the condition in some individuals. Additionally, deficiencies in certain nutrients, such as omega-3 fatty acids, may also increase the risk of developing ADHD.

5. Developmental Factors

Some researchers believe that developmental factors, such as delays in language and motor skills, may also contribute to the development of ADHD. Children who experience delays in these areas may have a higher risk of developing ADHD as they struggle to keep up with their peers.

In conclusion, ADHD is a complex condition, and while the causes are not entirely understood, it is clear that multiple factors may contribute to its development. Genetics, brain function, environmental factors, diet, and developmental factors can all play a role in increasing the risk of developing this condition. For individuals with ADHD, early diagnosis and treatment can significantly improve outcomes and quality of life.

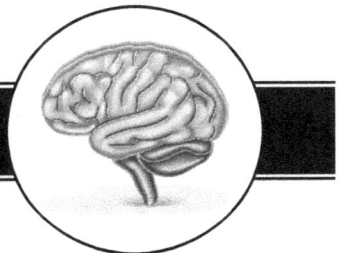

CHAPTER THREE

TYPES OF ADHD: INATTENTIVE, HYPERACTIVE, AND COMBINED

That is correct! ADHD (Attention-Deficit/Hyperactivity Disorder) can be classified into three types:

1. Inattentive Type - People with this type of ADHD have difficulty paying attention and staying focused on tasks. They are easily distracted and may struggle with organization and follow-through.

2. Hyperactive Type - People with this type of ADHD are hyperactive and have difficulty sitting still. They may have trouble controlling their impulses and may act impulsively or without thinking.

3. Combined Type - People with this type of ADHD have symptoms of both inattentiveness and hyperactivity. They may struggle with both attention and impulsivity.

It is important to note that ADHD presents differently in every individual, and some people may have symptoms that do not fit neatly into one of these categories. A professional diagnosis should always be sought if there are concerns about ADHD.

CHAPTER FOUR

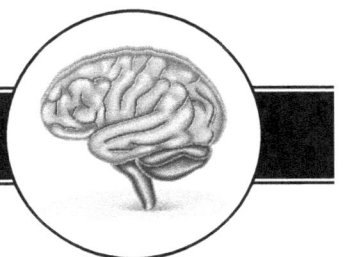

ADHD AND CO-EXISTING CONDITIONS: LEARNING DISABILITIES, ANXIETY, AND DEPRESSION

Attention-Deficit/Hyperactivity Disorder, commonly known as ADHD, is a neurodevelopmental disorder that affects people worldwide. ADHD is characterized by inattention, hyperactivity, and impulsivity which affects the individual's behavior and ability to focus.

Children and adults with ADHD often have co-existing conditions like learning disabilities, anxiety, and depression. In this article, we will explore the relationship between ADHD and co-existing conditions, specifically learning disabilities, anxiety, and depression.

Learning Disabilities:

Learning disabilities are common in children and adults with ADHD, affecting roughly 30% of individuals with the disorder. These disabilities can include challenges in reading, writing, and arithmetic. Learning disabilities result from differences in how the brain processes information, and often go undiagnosed and untreated in individuals with ADHD.

The cognitive difficulties associated with ADHD and Learning Disabilities can lead to academic and career setbacks. Children with ADHD often struggle with following instructions, managing time, paying attention, and organizing thoughts effectively. To address learning disabilities within ADHD, individuals may require additional support, such as accommodations at school or therapy focused on developing skills in areas that are challenging.

Anxiety:

Anxiety is a common co-existing condition in people with ADHD, impacting 25-40% of those with the disorder. Anxiety in individuals with ADHD can manifest in different ways, including social anxiety, obsessive-compulsive disorder, and generalized anxiety disorder.

It's essential to recognize that anxiety can exacerbate ADHD symptoms, causing intense mental and physical discomfort.

Individuals with ADHD and anxiety may worry excessively about assignments, their social interactions, and the future. The combination of ADHD and anxiety can affect self-esteem and lead to social isolation, which can impact social and academic growth negatively.

Depression:

Depression is a common co-existing condition in individuals with ADHD, and research suggests that approximately 50% of individuals with ADHD may experience depression. Some studies suggest several factors increase the risk of depression in individuals with ADHD, including poor self-esteem, struggling with school or work, and difficulties in social relationships.

Depression can exacerbate ADHD symptoms and impact daily life, such as difficulty sleeping and eating, low interest in activities, low mood, and feelings of hopelessness. Depression can decrease quality of life and can adversely affect academic and professional success at a young age.

In conclusion, individuals with ADHD frequently experience co-existing conditions, such as learning disabilities, anxiety, and depression. These conditions can complicate the treatment of ADHD and require additional support and intervention to mitigate their effects

Is autism and ADHD interlinked

Autism and ADHD, or attention deficit hyperactivity disorder, are two conditions that have been closely studied by medical professionals and researchers alike. While they may present with different symptoms, there is a growing body of evidence that suggests these two conditions are closely interlinked.

Autism, also known as autism spectrum disorder, is a developmental disorder that affects a person's ability to communicate, socialize, and interact with others. It is characterized by repetitive behaviors, difficulties with social interaction, and restricted interests. ADHD, on the other hand, is a neurodevelopmental disorder that affects a person's ability to focus, sit still, and control their impulses.

Studies have shown that there is a high degree of comorbidity, or co-occurrence, between autism and ADHD. According to one study, approximately 30-50% of individuals with autism also have ADHD, and vice versa. This suggests that there may be underlying genetic or environmental factors that contribute to the development of both conditions.

One of the reasons why autism and ADHD are thought to be linked is that they share many common symptoms. For example, difficulties with social interaction, impulsivity, and hyperactivity are all features that can be present in both conditions. It is not uncommon for individuals with autism to also struggle with attention and focus, which are hallmark features of ADHD.

In addition, certain medications that are commonly used to treat ADHD, such as stimulant medications like Adderall and Ritalin, have also been found to be effective in improving symptoms of autism. This further supports the idea that there may be shared underlying mechanisms between these two conditions.

With that being said, it is important to note that not all individuals with autism or ADHD will have both conditions. Each person is unique, and their experiences and symptoms may differ. However, overall, the evidence suggests that there is a close link between these two conditions.

To give some specific examples, imagine a child who has been diagnosed with autism. This child may struggle with social interaction, repetitive behaviors, and intense fixation on certain interests. Over time, it becomes apparent that they also have difficulty staying focused in class and are easily distracted. Upon further evaluation, they may be diagnosed with ADHD as well.

On the flipside, a child who has been diagnosed with ADHD may have difficulty controlling their impulses and sitting still, and may struggle with following social norms and rules. Over time, it becomes apparent that they also have difficulty with reading social cues and understanding the nuances of social interaction

ADHD and Sleep difficulties

Attention Deficit Hyperactivity Disorder (ADHD) is a neurodevelopmental disorder that affects both children and adults. It is characterized by symptoms such as inattention, hyperactivity, and impulsivity. As a result, it can have a significant impact on everyday life, including sleep patterns. In this blog, we will explore the link between ADHD and sleep difficulties, and provide tips on how to improve sleep quality.

One of the main symptoms of ADHD is hyperactivity, which can make it difficult to fall asleep at night. Individuals with ADHD may also have racing thoughts, which can further interfere with sleep onset. Moreover, the inattentiveness associated with ADHD can lead to poor time management, resulting in an irregular sleep schedule.

Sleep difficulties can exacerbate ADHD symptoms, as lack of sleep can lead to increased symptoms of inattention, irritability, and impulsivity. Therefore, it is crucial to establish healthy sleep habits and develop strategies to improve sleep quality.

Here are some tips that can help individuals with ADHD improve their sleep patterns:

1. Establish a Sleep Routine: Developing a consistent sleep routine can help regulate the body's internal clock and improve sleep efficiency. It is recommended to go to bed and wake up at the same time every day, including weekends.

2. Create a Sleep-conducive Environment: Ensure that the sleep environment is comfortable, quiet, and dark. Avoiding stimulating activities such as using electronics and engaging in mentally stimulating activities before bedtime.

3. Implement Relaxation Techniques: Relaxation techniques such as meditation, deep breathing, and progressive muscle relaxation can help calm the mind and body, making it easier to fall asleep.

4. Regular Exercise: Regular exercise during the day can aid in the regulation of the sleep-wake cycle and improve sleep quality. However, it is advisable to avoid exercising close to bedtime.

5. Avoid Stimulants: Avoid consuming stimulants such as caffeine, nicotine, and alcohol close to bedtime, as they can hinder the ability to fall asleep.

6. Seek Professional Help: Professionals like counselors, therapists, or sleep specialists can provide support and guidance in changing sleep patterns and other ADHD-related symptoms.

In conclusion, ADHD and sleep difficulties can be challenging to manage. However, developing healthy sleep habits and seeking support from a professional can hugely impact one's quality of life. With these tips provided above, individuals with ADHD can learn to manage their sleep difficulties and develop better sleep patterns, which will ultimately lead to healthier and more productive lives.

ADHD and Emotional Dysregulation

ADHD (Attention Deficit Hyperactivity Disorder) is a neurodevelopmental disorder that affects the ability to pay attention, focus, and manage time. Emotional dysregulation is a symptom that often occurs in individuals with ADHD, which is characterized by difficulty regulating and expressing emotions appropriately.

Real-life examples of emotional dysregulation in individuals with ADHD can include:

1. Intense reactions: People with ADHD can be prone to overreacting to situations, getting very upset or angry. For example, getting upset over minor inconveniences, like a missed appointment or a small mistake.

2. Impulsivity: Individuals with ADHD may act impulsively without thinking the consequences through. For example, speaking out in class without raising their hand or interrupting others during conversations.

3. Difficulty regulating emotions: Individuals with ADHD may struggle to control their emotions, leading to outbursts or meltdowns. For example, feeling overwhelmed and crying in public, or getting angry over minor things.

4. Quick mood changes: Individuals with ADHD may experience rapid mood swings and have trouble regulating their emotions. For example, feeling very happy one moment and then becoming angry or sad the next moment.

5. Sensitivity to criticism: Individuals with ADHD might be sensitive to criticism and react strongly to perceived negative feedback. For example, becoming defensive or feeling significantly downhearted after receiving negative feedback.

It's important to note that not everyone with ADHD experiences emotional dysregulation and those who experience may not experience it in the exact same way. It's best to work with a healthcare professional who can give guidance and support in managing these symptoms.

CHAPTER FIVE

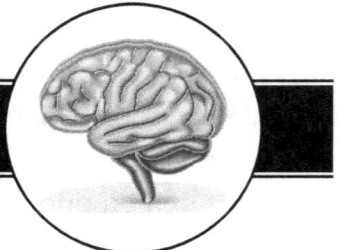

TREATMENT OPTIONS FOR ADHD: MEDICATIONS, THERAPY, AND LIFESTYLE CHANGES

Before we go in to this topic let me try and give you some guidance regarding the following -How to explain ADHD to my child

Explaining ADHD to a child as a parent can be a tough task, but with the right approach and language, it can help them understand themselves better. Here is a detailed plan that can help you explain ADHD to your child:

1. Introduce the concept of ADHD in simple language.
Start by explaining that there is a condition called ADHD that some people have, which can make it hard for them to stay focused or sit still. Reinforce the idea that it is a common thing and that many people have it.

2. Describe how ADHD affects their behavior.

Explain that having ADHD can make things like following instructions, finishing tasks, and keeping their attention on one thing difficult. You can ask them if they have ever experienced these things and explain that it has nothing to do with their intelligence or ability to learn.

3. Give them examples to help them understand.

Giving examples of situations where they've found it hard to focus or stay still can help your child understand how ADHD works. For example, you can talk about when they were playing a game and found it hard to stick to the rules or when they had trouble paying attention during class.

4. Discuss treatment options.

Once your child understands ADHD, it's important to discuss what can be done to help. Explain different treatment options such as medication, therapy, and lifestyle changes, and emphasize how all of them can help manage their ADHD symptoms.

5. Encourage them to ask questions.

It's important to create an open environment where your child feels comfortable asking questions. Encourage them to share their thoughts and feelings about ADHD, so you can help them navigate through their condition.

Overall, the most important thing when explaining ADHD to your child is to highlight the fact that it's not a sign of weakness or inability. Help your child understand that ADHD is simply a part of who they are, and that it's nothing to be ashamed of. By being supportive and understanding, you'll provide the tools they need to manage their ADHD symptoms and to succeed in life.

Attention Deficit Hyperactivity Disorder (ADHD) is a common neurodevelopmental disorder that affects both children and adults. According to the National Institute of Mental Health, approximately 6.1 million children between the ages of 2 and 17 have been diagnosed with ADHD in the United States.

ADHD can be challenging for both the individuals affected and those around them. Medications can help manage symptoms and improve daily functioning. In this article, we will discuss the different types of medications available for ADHD and how they work.

Stimulants are the most commonly prescribed medications for ADHD. They work by increasing the neurotransmitters dopamine and norepinephrine, which help improve attention, focus, and impulse control. Stimulants are available in both short-acting and long-acting forms.

Short-acting stimulants, like Ritalin and Adderall, typically last for around four hours and may need to be taken multiple times a day. Long-acting stimulants, like Concerta and Vyvanse, last anywhere from 8 to 12 hours and only need to be taken once a day.

Another type of medication for ADHD is non-stimulant medications. These medications work by targeting different neurotransmitters to help improve attention and reduce hyperactivity. Non-stimulant medications include Strattera and Intuniv. Strattera is a selective norepinephrine reuptake inhibitor (SNRI), which means it increases the levels of norepinephrine in the brain. Intuniv is an alpha-2 agonist, which helps to reduce hyperactivity and impulsivity.

In addition to medication, it's important to have a comprehensive treatment plan for ADHD, which may include therapy, lifestyle changes, and behavior modifications. Medications alone are not a cure for ADHD, but they can be an effective tool in managing symptoms.

It's also important to note that medication may not be the best option for every child with ADHD. Each child responds differently to medication, and some may experience side effects. It's essential to work closely with a healthcare provider to determine the best course of treatment.

In conclusion, medication can be an essential tool in managing ADHD symptoms for children and adults. Stimulants and non-stimulant medications work by targeting different neurotransmitters in the brain to help improve attention, focus, and impulse control. It's important to have a comprehensive treatment plan for ADHD that includes therapy, lifestyle changes, and behavior modifications in addition.

Therapies for ADHD

Here are five therapies that have been found to be effective in managing ADHD symptoms:

1. Behavioral therapy: This therapy focuses on teaching individuals with ADHD how to change their behavior through positive reinforcement and structure. Behavioral therapy provides practical strategies to manage symptoms, such as keeping a schedule and breaking down tasks into smaller, more manageable steps. The goal is to help individuals with ADHD develop more effective coping mechanisms and improve their functioning in daily life.

2. Cognitive-behavioral therapy (CBT): CBT focuses on the thoughts and beliefs that influence behavior. This therapy helps individuals with ADHD identify negative thoughts and replace them with positive ones. This technique can help individuals with ADHD develop skills to manage stress, impulsivity, and decision-making skills.

3. Mindfulness meditation: This practice helps individuals with ADHD become more aware of their thoughts and emotions.

Mindfulness meditation teaches individuals to focus on the present moment and reduce distractions. People with ADHD may find that mindfulness meditation increases their attention span, reduces impulsivity, and enhances cognitive flexibility.

4. Neurofeedback: Neurofeedback uses visual and auditory feedback to train individuals' brains to regulate their brain waves. In neurofeedback, individuals wear EEG sensors that measure their brain activity. This technique helps individuals learn to control their brain waves, which can improve focus, attention, and reduce impulsivity.

5. Exercise: Exercise is another non-medication therapy that has been shown to be helpful for individuals with ADHD. Exercise can help individuals with ADHD by reducing stress, increasing dopamine and norepinephrine levels in the brain, improving sleep, and enhancing cognitive function.

Overall, these therapies aim to help individuals with ADHD improve their focus, reduce impulsivity, and develop effective coping strategies. These therapies offer drug-free alternatives to manage ADHD symptoms and improve overall functioning.

Lifestyle changes in kids with ADHD

Attention Deficit Hyperactivity Disorder (ADHD) is a neurodevelopmental disorder affecting millions of children worldwide. ADHD is a complex disorder characterized by inattention, hyperactivity, and impulsiveness. Children with ADHD can have difficulty focusing, completing tasks, and following instructions. These challenges can cause stress and frustration for both the child and their family.

Fortunately, parents and caregivers can help manage ADHD symptoms by making lifestyle changes. These changes can improve a child's quality of life while reducing their ADHD symptoms.

1. Encourage a healthy diet
The brain needs a balanced diet to function properly, and children with ADHD may benefit from certain foods. Encourage your child to eat a balanced diet with plenty of fruits, vegetables, lean proteins and whole grains. Avoid processed foods and sugary snacks as they can cause sugar crashes that can worsen ADHD symptoms.

2. Get enough sleep
Getting enough sleep is essential for children with ADHD. Sleep deprivation can increase symptoms of inattention and hyperactivity. Set a regular sleep schedule and make sure your child gets enough sleep every night.

3. Create a routine
Children with ADHD benefit from structure and routine. A consistent daily routine can help with their behavior and emotional regulation. Creating a structured schedule for activities like eating, sleeping, and studying can positively impact a child's ADHD symptoms.

4. Physical activity
Physical activity is essential for improving ADHD symptoms as it improves focus and concentration. Encourage your child to take up an active hobby or sport. For example, playing soccer, riding a bike or swimming can help to reduce hyperactivity and increase focus.

5. Mindfulness
Mindfulness can be a helpful technique for children with ADHD to manage their symptoms. Mindfulness exercises involve focusing on physical sensations, the breath, and thoughts. It has been found that mindfulness meditation practice can help children with ADHD to better manage their symptoms.

6. Limit screen time
Limiting screen time can be challenging in our modern world, but it is an essential part of managing ADHD symptoms. Too much screen time can distract children from other activities or create further mental stimulation that can interfere with their sleep patterns.

7. Social skills

Teaching social skills is also essential for children with ADHD. For example, encourage your child to participate in activities with other children or join clubs that focus on their interests. Practising social skills can help to reduce feelings of social isolation, and gain confidence and a sense of belonging.

In conclusion, ADHD can be challenging, but lifestyle changes can significantly alter the outlook of your child's ADHD difficulties

Behaviour modification strategies for ADHD

ADHD, which stands for Attention Deficit Hyperactivity Disorder, is a condition affecting children's behaviour, making them impulsive, hyperactive, and having difficulty paying attention. Managing the behaviour of children with ADHD can be overwhelming for parents, teachers, and caregivers. Behaviour modification strategies are effective coping mechanisms that have been successfully used to manage ADHD in children.

Here are some behaviour modification strategies to help kids with ADHD and help parents:

1. Positive reinforcement: This involves recognizing and rewarding good behaviour. Praising and rewarding kids for desired behaviour enhances their sense of accomplishment and promotes positive reinforcement. For example, you can praise your child for finishing their homework or for sitting quietly during dinner time.

2. Consistency: Consistent rules and routines can help children with ADHD know what to expect and understand the consequences of their actions. This can improve their ability to regulate their behaviour and stay in control. For instance, having a consistent bedtime routine can help children relax and prepare for sleep.

3. Clear communication: Children with ADHD often struggle with processing information. Simple language and clear communication can improve their understanding and reduce confusion. Using specific instructions and visual aids can also help to reinforce the message. For example, having a checklist for daily tasks like getting dressed or brushing teeth can help kids with ADHD stay organized.

4. Time management: Children with ADHD often have trouble managing their time and staying focused on a task. Breaking down larger tasks into smaller ones and making use of timers can help them stay on track. Parents can also help by setting realistic expectations for their child's completion of tasks.

5. Exercise: Exercise is a great way to reduce hyperactivity and improve focus. Encouraging your child to participate in physical activities like sports or bike riding can improve their ability to focus and reduce impulsive behaviour.

6. Mindfulness: Mindfulness techniques can help children with ADHD manage their emotions and stay calm. Practising mindful breathing, guided meditation or progressive muscle relaxation can help them feel more relaxed and less stressed.

In summary, ADHD in children can be managed effectively with the above behaviour modification strategies. Consistency, clear communication, positive reinforcement, exercise, time management, and mindfulness are techniques that parents can use to help their child cope effectively with ADHD symptoms.

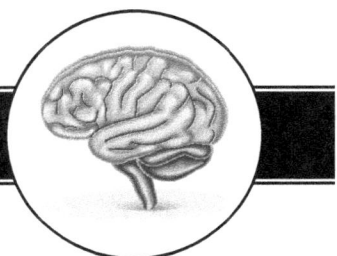

CHAPTER SIX

PARENTING A CHILD WITH ADHD: STRATEGIES FOR MANAGING BEHAVIOR AND IMPROVING COMMUNICATION

1. Understand what ADHD is and how it affects your child's behavior

2. Consult with a doctor or therapist to determine the best course of treatment for your child

3. Create a consistent routine and structure for your child

4. Use positive reinforcement to encourage good behavior

5. Set goals and rewards for your child's progress

6. Use visual aids and schedules to help your child stay organized and focused

7. Provide a distraction-free environment for your child to do homework or other tasks

8. Use short and clear instructions when communicating with your child

9. Practice active listening and empathy when communicating with your child

10. Teach your child self-regulation techniques such as deep breathing or mindfulness

11. Break down tasks into smaller steps to make them more manageable for your child

12. Encourage physical activity and exercise to help your child release energy and reduce symptoms

13. Limit screen time and other stimulating activities before bedtime to improve sleep quality

14. Collaborate with your child's school to develop a plan for academic accommodations and support

15. Seek out parent support groups or online forums to connect with other parents in similar situations

16. Take care of your own mental and physical health to better support your child

17. Develop strategies for handling behavior outbursts or other challenging situations

18. Encourage your child's passions and interests to boost their self-esteem and confidence

19. Be patient and persistent in implementing strategies and seeking progress

20. Celebrate your child's successes and growth, no matter how small.

How to manage my child's self esteem
I have included this as it's a common question parents ask me about how to manage my child's self esteem

Managing low self-esteem in a child with ADHD can be challenging, but there are some strategies that parents and caregivers can use to help the child feel more confident and positive about themselves. Here are some tips:

1. Acknowledge their strengths: Children with ADHD often struggle with negative feedback and criticism. Therefore, it is crucial to acknowledge their strengths and positive behaviors. Encourage and praise them for their successes, no matter how small.

2. Set achievable goals: Set small, achievable goals that are specific, realistic, and measurable. This helps the child gain a sense of achievement and boosts their confidence.

3. Encourage socializing: Encourage the child to socialize with peers who have similar interests, as this helps them feel accepted and valued by others.

4. Focus on positive self-talk: Teach the child to practice positive self-talk by replacing negative, self-critical thoughts with positive affirmations. For instance, instead of saying, "I am dumb," encourage them to say, "I am capable of learning."

5. Seek professional help: Consider seeking the help of a therapist or counselor who specializes in ADHD to help the child manage their symptoms and improve their self-esteem.

CHAPTER SEVEN

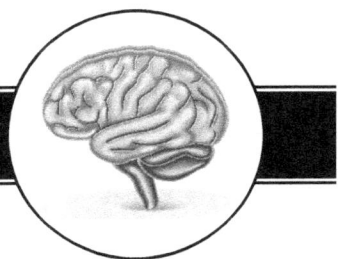

ADHD IN SCHOOL: ACCOMMODATIONS AND SUPPORT FOR ACADEMIC SUCCESS

Here are 30 different points on accommodating and supporting academic success for students with ADHD in school:

1. Provide the student with a quiet, private space for studying and taking tests.

2. Allow the student to take breaks as necessary to manage hyperactivity.

3. Provide multi-sensory materials (such as audio or visual aids) to help with focus and attention.

4. Break down assignments into smaller, manageable tasks.

5. Allow for flexibility in due dates for assignments.

6. Provide prompts or reminders for when assignments are due.

7. Implement a behavior management plan to address disruptive behaviors.

8. Use positive reinforcement for desired behaviors.

9. Provide feedback to the student on their progress.

10. Use graphic organizers to help with organization and planning.

11. Provide access to assistive technology, such as speech-to-text software.

12. Limit distractions in the classroom as much as possible.

13. Provide opportunities for physical movement in the classroom.

14. Encourage the use of fidget toys or stress balls to release energy.

15. Use color-coding or other visual aids to help with organization and memory.

16. Provide the option to take shorter quizzes or assessments.

17. Allow the student to listen to music using headphones as long as it is not too distracting.

18. Encourage the student to use study groups or peer support networks.

19. Offer additional support from a school counselor or social worker.

20. Provide daily or weekly schedules to help with planning and organization.

21. Use frequent, short breaks throughout the day to help with managing attention.

22. Encourage the student to write down important information and instructions.

23. Offer tutoring or extra help sessions.

24. Provide opportunities for the student to move around during class.

25. Use visual timers to help the student stay on task.

26. Encourage the use of agenda books or planner apps.

27. Offer alternative testing formats, such as oral exams.

28. Provide positive feedback for effort and improvement, not just achievement.

29. Communicate regularly with parents and caregivers about the student's progress.

30. Educate other students and teachers about ADHD to reduce stigma and increase understanding.

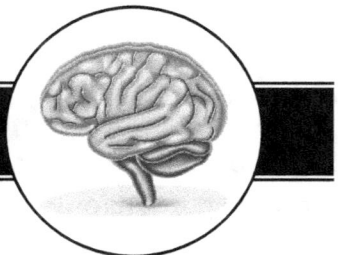

CHAPTER EIGHT

SOCIAL SKILLS AND ADHD: HELPING CHILDREN MAKE AND KEEP FRIENDS

Attention deficit hyperactivity disorder (ADHD) can have a significant impact on a child's social skills, making it challenging for them to make and keep friends. As a parent or caregiver, you can help children with ADHD develop social skills that will enable them to fit in and form meaningful relationships with their peers.

Here are some tips for helping children with ADHD develop social skills:

1. Teach basic social skills: Basic social skills like sharing, taking turns, and saying please and thank you are essential to building healthy relationships. Teach and reinforce these skills consistently, and provide positive feedback when children display them.

2. Practice conversational skills: Conversational skills like asking questions, listening attentively, and taking turns talking can be challenging for children with ADHD. Encourage children to practice these skills during play dates and other social activities. Role-playing and creating scripts can also be helpful.

3. Encourage empathy: Children with ADHD can struggle to understand other people's feelings and perspectives. Empathy is a critical component of building relationships. Encourage children to put themselves in other people's shoes, and teach them to recognize and respond to others' emotions.

4. Promote self-awareness: Children with ADHD often struggle with impulse control and emotional regulation, which can impact their social interactions. Help them develop self-awareness by encouraging them to reflect on their behavior and feelings. You can also teach them mindfulness practices that help them observe their thoughts and feelings without judgment.

5. Provide opportunities for social interaction: Children with ADHD may struggle with social situations, but they need opportunities to practice and refine their social skills. Encourage participation in group activities and clubs, and provide opportunities for play dates and other social outings.

Examples:

1. Role-playing: Practice social situations with your child by role-playing scenarios like introducing themselves to someone new, asking for a turn, or resolving a conflict with a friend.

2. Empathy exercises: Play games that help children recognize facial expressions and emotions, and encourage them to respond appropriately.

3. Group activities: Encourage your child to participate in group activities like sports, clubs, or music lessons, where they can practice their social skills in a structured environment.

4. Play dates: Host play dates with classmates or friends, and provide activities that promote socialization, like board games, crafts, or outdoor play.

In conclusion, helping children with ADHD develop social skills is critical to their overall wellbeing and success in life. By teaching basic social skills, practicing conversation skills, promoting self awareness will all help your child to have a better social life and ultimately be happy about themselves.

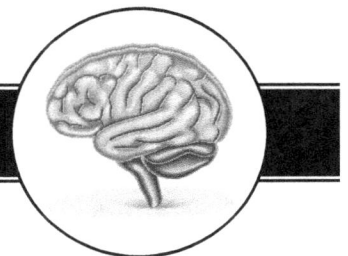

CHAPTER NINE

ADHD AND FAMILY RELATIONSHIPS: MAINTAINING A POSITIVE AND SUPPORTIVE HOME ENVIRONMENT

Here is a detailed plan on how to maintain a positive and supportive home environment for someone with ADHD and their family:

1. Establish clear expectations and routines: People with ADHD thrive in structured environments. Establishing clear expectations and sticking to routines can help them understand what is expected of them and reduce their stress levels. For example, you can create a set schedule for meals, daily chores, and homework time.

2. Set clear communication channels: Communication can be a challenge for people with ADHD, so it's important to establish clear communication channels. You can do this by:

- Establishing non-verbal communication signals when you need their attention.
- Setting up weekly family meetings to discuss upcoming events, concerns, and expectations.
- Use a whiteboard in a central location to keep everyone updated on what's happening in the household.

3. Encourage self-care practices: People with ADHD can easily become overwhelmed and stressed out. Encouraging self-care practices, such as exercise or meditation, can help them manage their symptoms. For example, you can encourage your family member to take daily walks or practice mindfulness exercises.

4. Foster a judgment-free environment: Having ADHD can be challenging, and individuals with ADHD can be their worst critics. Creating a judgment-free environment where everyone feels accepted and comfortable can be a game-changer. For example, you can avoid making harsh or sarcastic comments about their forgetfulness or impulsivity.

5. Have open and honest communication: Encouraging open and honest communication can help family members with ADHD feel heard and understood. You can achieve this by:

- Asking open-ended questions that invite conversation and expression of feelings.

- Using active listening techniques, such as paraphrasing and clarifying, to show that you understand their viewpoint.
- Avoiding interrupting or dismissing their feelings.

6. Be flexible and adaptable: Finally, it's important to be flexible and adaptable when it comes to your family member's needs. ADHD symptoms can vary from day to day, so being able to adjust routines and expectations can make a big difference. For example, if your family member is having a particularly challenging day, you can adjust their schedule to allow for more breaks or rest periods.

Overall, maintaining a positive and supportive home environment for someone with ADHD requires understanding, patience, and flexibility. With these strategies in place, you can create an environment that helps your family member thrive.

CHAPTER TEN

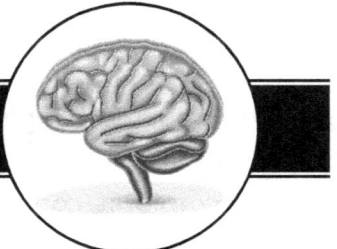

COPING WITH ADHD AS A FAMILY: ADVICE FOR MANAGING STRESS, STAYING MOTIVATED, AND CELEBRATING PROGRESS.

Sure, here is an article that you might find helpful:

Coping with ADHD as a Family: Advice for Managing Stress, Staying Motivated, and Celebrating Progress

Attention Deficit Hyperactivity Disorder (ADHD) is a neurodevelopmental disorder that affects both children and adults. It can create challenges for individuals with ADHD as well as their families. However, with a little knowledge, understanding, and support, managing ADHD can become easier. Here are some tips for coping with ADHD as a family.

1. Maintain a Regular Schedule

It is essential to follow a steady routine, especially for individuals with ADHD. A predictable schedule allows them to manage their time better, be less prone to procrastination, and develop healthy habits.

For instance, if the family follows a morning routine to get ready for school or work, stick to it. Post the schedule in the common area of the house, and make sure each family member knows his or her role in following the routine.

2. Minimize Distractions

Individuals with ADHD often have trouble concentrating due to distractions. Therefore, it is crucial to create an environment that is conducive to focus. Turn off the television, limit access to electronic devices, and create a quiet space to work.

For example, set aside time for homework or any other focused tasks, and try to limit noise or other stimuli that can be distracting. In addition, during meal times, try to have a technology-free zone to avoid any distractions.

3. Emphasize the Positive

It is important to create a positive environment and emphasize achievements rather than shortcomings. Recognize the strengths of each family member and highlight them.

For example, if your child gets good grades, praise their efforts and hard work. If a task seems impossible, break it down into smaller steps, and celebrate each milestone.

4. Encourage Exercise and Outdoor Activities

Individuals with ADHD often have excess energy and can become restless if they stay indoors for too long. Encourage physical activity and outdoor time, as it can help them release that extra energy and improve focus.

For instance, make it a habit to go for a family walk after dinner, sign-up for a sports program, or make sure there is an outdoor area available where your child can play.

5. Create a Support System

Get support from family, friends, school, or therapists who understand ADHD. Seek guidance and advice when necessary.

For example, try to attend support sessions or seek counseling to stay informed about ADHD.

How do support groups help for adhd managment

Support groups can be very helpful for both parents and children who are dealing with ADHD. Here are some ways that support groups can help in managing your child's ADHD:

1. Education: Many support groups provide information about the latest research on ADHD, as well as resources for managing symptoms.

2. Peer support: Children with ADHD can benefit greatly from meeting peers who are facing similar challenges. This can help them feel less alone and isolated.

3. Parenting strategies: Support groups often provide tips and strategies for parents on how to manage their child's ADHD, such as behavior modification techniques and medication management.

4. Coping skills: Support groups can also provide coping skills for both parents and children, such as mindfulness exercises and stress reduction techniques.

Overall, support groups can provide a valuable community for families dealing with ADHD, and can help everyone involved feel more supported and informed.

MYTHS ABOUT ADHD

Sure, here are ten common myths about ADHD and the actual truth, supported by research:

Myth #1: ADHD isn't a real disorder.

Truth: ADHD is a well-established disorder with a clear set of diagnostic criteria. It is recognized as a legitimate disorder by the American Psychiatric Association, the World Health Organization, and other major medical and mental health authorities.

Myth #2: ADHD only affects children.

Truth: ADHD is often first diagnosed in childhood, but it can persist into adulthood. In fact, estimates suggest that up to 60% of children with ADHD will continue to have symptoms into adulthood.

Myth #3: ADHD is caused by bad parenting or lack of discipline.

Truth: ADHD is a neurodevelopmental disorder with a strong genetic component. While parenting style and environmental factors may impact symptom severity, they do not cause ADHD.

Myth #4: ADHD only affects boys.

Truth: While it's true that boys are more likely to be diagnosed with ADHD than girls, this may be due to diagnostic bias rather than an actual gender difference in prevalence. Girls with ADHD are often overlooked because they may present differently than boys, exhibiting less hyperactive behavior.

Myth #5: Medication is the only effective treatment for ADHD.

Truth: While medication can be an effective treatment for ADHD, it is not the only option. Behavioral therapy, coaching, and lifestyle changes (such as exercise, a healthy diet, and good sleep hygiene) can also be helpful.

Myth #6: People with ADHD can't pay attention to anything.

Truth: While attention deficits are a hallmark of ADHD, people with the disorder can focus intently on things that interest them. The challenge is maintaining focus on less stimulating tasks.

Myth #7: People with ADHD are lazy or unmotivated.

Truth: People with ADHD often struggle with motivation and organization, but this is not due to laziness or lack of willpower. It's a result of neurological differences in the brain that affect executive functioning.

Myth #8: People with ADHD can't succeed in school or in their careers.

Truth: While ADHD can make academic and professional success more challenging, many people with the disorder have successful careers and fulfilling lives with proper treatment and accommodations.

Myth #9: ADHD is overdiagnosed and overmedicated.

Truth: While there may be some instances of overdiagnosis and overmedication, research suggests that ADHD is still under-recognized and undertreated.

HERE ARE TEN FACTS ABOUT ADHD THAT KIDS MAY FIND INTERESTING AND HELPFUL:

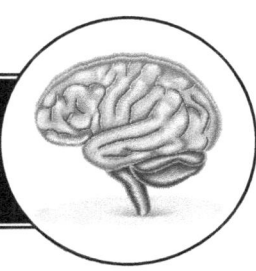

1. Some people with ADHD have what's called "hyperfocus," where they become extremely absorbed in a task they enjoy and can lose track of time.

2. ADHD affects both boys and girls and people with ADHD come from all racial, ethnic, and socioeconomic backgrounds.

3. Some famous people with ADHD include Michael Phelps, Justin Timberlake, and Simone Biles.

4. People with ADHD are often great at thinking outside the box and coming up with creative solutions.

5. ADHD is not caused by bad parenting or too much sugar.

6. Medication can be helpful for some people with ADHD, but it's not the only treatment option.

7. Exercise can be a great way to help manage ADHD symptoms, as it can help with focus and attention.

8. People with ADHD may struggle with impulsivity, but with practice and patience, they can learn how to pause and think before acting.

9. ADHD is not a measure of intelligence or potential. Many people with ADHD go on to be successful in their careers and personal lives.

10. Having ADHD is just one part of who a person is -- they are also kind, creative, funny, and many other wonderful things!

www.ingramcontent.com/pod-product-compliance
Lightning Source LLC
Chambersburg PA
CBHW070438290526
45791CB00005B/2035